"The same thought kept occurring to me or 'It's real. These are true feelings.' It is comforting to know that God is the way, truth, and life eternal. Peppered throughout the pages I see the feelings of peace that all people search for while here on earth."

Madeline Tetrault

"Donna's inspirational book has provided me with an excellent resource for confronting the challenges of living with a chronic illness. God Bless you, Donna."

Constance (Connie) Hoyack.

"Priceless. Honest. Uplifting. A true testimony to walking in faith, not by sight."

Constance James

"This book is extraordinary. My mother had a chronic illness and neither of us handled it very well. The problem was communication and understanding each other. I believe that with this book, I could have reached out with the power of prayer and something in common, to help her through the difficult times."

Dorthea R. Stanhope

"Inspiring, comforting meditations for the chronically ill that will help a suffering person through even the worst days."

Pam Bass

"Chronic illness is a tough and lonely process for many. Donna J. Coble has written meditations that will help the lonely ones to cope."

Beverly Evans

"Sometimes with chronic illness, the answers for *why* we are sick are not there. This book is definitely a good start."

Judith M. Fox

So you have a chronic illness?

So you have a chronic illness?

WHAT NOW?

Donna J. Coble

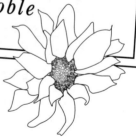

Published by Tate Publishing & Enterprises, LLC
127 E. Trade Center Terrace | Mustang, Oklahoma 73064 USA
1.888.361.9473 | www.tatepublishing.com

Tate Publishing is committed to excellence in the publishing industry. The company reflects the philosophy established by the founders, based on Psalm 68:11,
"The Lord gave the word and great was the company of those who published it."

Book design copyright © 2008 by Tate Publishing, LLC. All rights reserved.
Cover design by Leah LeFlore
Interior design by Melanie Harr-Hughes

Published in the United States of America

ISBN: 978-1-60604-630-2
1. Health & fitness / diseases / general
2. Biography & autobiography / medical
08.10.21

This book is dedicated to Bob Coble,
my loving husband of over fifty years.

Acknowledgments

I give thanks for God's inspiration and to my family and friends for their encouragement.

CONTENTS

Foreword

I had the privilege to meet Donna Coble two years ago. She was a delightful but frail woman confined to her wheelchair. She had trouble enunciating her words, but with considerable effort she could clearly make herself understood, and we had a delightful conversation. I was impressed by this intelligent woman. Her bright eyes reflected a vibrant and active mind—a person with much to share. We spent over an hour talking about our love of God and Jesus Christ. Despite her obvious disability, she was a joy to behold.

Several months later I invited Donna and her husband, Bob, to come to our church where she presented her first book, *A Family's Daily Devotional for a Year*. With amplification her soft voice could be heard, and this petite woman captivated our congregation with her love of God. At the book signing most of the church bought Donna's book.

In Donna's second book, *So You Have A Chronic Illness… What Now?*, Donna writes about her own illness. I was touched by her complete honesty revealing her disability with candor, showing her daily struggles with this disease and with her own human limitations.

With any progressive, unrelenting illness, each day is a challenge—a battle to accomplish even the simplest of tasks. Donna describes her own battle with fatigue, pain, insomnia, isolation, anger, loneliness, dependency, and depression. We would all feel this way while struggling with a chronic disease. It is relatively easy for a healthy person to say "I will stay positive" or "I will overcome this hardship," but it is a very difficult thing to do for someone with a chronic illness. For these patients, health victories are measured when symptoms slightly abate.

Donna didn't write this book to chronicle her disease but to show the great hope one can have by staying close to God. It is not a self-help work or one showing techniques to help with the disease; rather, it teaches to rely ever more on God, His strength, and

His revealed understanding. Donna presents a genuine attempt to daily surrender to God in the hope of coping better and finding personal peace. "Blessed are the peace makers for they will be called the sons (and daughters) of God" (Matthew 5:9, KJV). Donna is definitely such a peacemaker and an inspiration.

No one wants to think that one day they will have to deal with a chronic illness. I know I don't. Unfortunately, in the future, millions of us will come down with a progressive chronic disease and, like Donna, will have to personally come to terms with this fact.

If this happens to me, I pray that I have the insight and stamina to do exactly as Donna has shown in her book, to rely on God and Christ as my strength. Donna Coble is a treasure. As Jesus said,

"These things I have spoken to you, that in Me you may have peace. In the world you will have tribulation; but be of good cheer, I have overcome the world" (John 16:33–17:1, NKJV).

I hope Donna Coble's book will help you to find peace.

Glenn R. Edgecombe, M. D.

Introduction

What is the definition of the word *chronic?* "Long-lasting: describes an illness or medical condition that lasts over a long period and sometimes causes a long-term change in the body."[1]

It all started when I was cleaning my brick porch. I fell backwards and fractured my left wrist. Over a period of time I had a number of falls. Then I noticed that I wasn't swinging my arms when I was walking. My arms and legs generally ached, and I felt stiff. I was terribly tired all the time. My left side grew weaker than the right side. It was harder to get dressed, as putting on a sweater, putting on my slacks, putting on my socks, and buttoning my clothes are nearly impossible to do with one hand. My doctor put me on a medication that made me nauseated for about three weeks. I finally adjusted to it. The medicine helped a little bit.

I had the usual tests, like Cat Scans and MRIs. Over time I grew worse. I started needing to have to use a walker because my balance was so bad. I had trouble talking. My voice was soft, and I couldn't pronounce my words. I was having trouble swallowing my food, and I was choking a lot. I now had balance problems so bad that I had—and still do—to use a wheelchair and power chair. I saw a neurologist, who said that I have Multiple System Atrophy. While it has some symptoms like Parkinson's, I don't have the shaking or tremor.

I find that not being able to talk clearly is my hardest thing to deal with; it limits socializing. Next is not being able to walk. I can still dress myself but not much else. I can't write in long hand. I can use the computer by hunting and pecking.

As time went on I got worse. I turned my illness over to God, a steadying force in my life. My husband and children have been wonderful. I know it is hard for them to watch my body succumb to this illness.

I have divided up this journal into six sections

corresponding with the six stages of chronic illness. The first one is being Sick and not knowing why. A person sometimes goes from test to test, specialist to specialist, and sometimes to emergency rooms and to hospital stays. Finally at long last the Diagnosis is made. You have a chronic illness. What a shock. You feel numb. You can't believe such a thing is happening to you. You begin to feel intense Anger. You ask yourself what caused the illness. What did I do? Did the doctor overlook something? Is God punishing me? Why me? You end up with a Depression. You feel sad. You don't feel interested in anything. You are so tired and have no energy. Then you come to the point that you are either going to sink or swim. And you decide to swim. You learn to Cope and work around your illness. At last you become adjusted to the change the illness has brought on. Your life is not the same. With God's grace you find peace in your heart. You learn that Acceptance and Hope are the only things that will keep you going.

Stage 1: Sick

New Year

Matthew 28:20 "Teach these new disciples to obey all the commands I have given you. And be sure of this: I am with you always, even to the end of the age."

Last year was a great year with a lot of spiritual growth. Reading Scripture everyday is wonderful. This time of quiet allows me time to think about the verse and my life. It makes the Scripture become real and alive.

God, I have had many problems to cope with this year. I feel ill. I don't know what is wrong with me. I have fallen down a lot lately. I lose my balance very easily. I don't seem to be swinging my arms when I am walking anymore. I feel stiff, and my muscles are sore. Most of all,

I feel very tired. It is hard to get through each day. Help me trust you that everything will be okay. Thank you.

➣ Have you ever had a year when everything seemed to go wrong?

_____

_____

_____

➣ How did you manage?

_____

_____

_____

Faith

Psalm 118:8–9 "It is better to trust the Lord than to put confidence in people. It is better to trust the Lord than to put confidence in princes."

I went over to a friend's house this afternoon, and I talked my head off about my problem I was having with my health. I talked about all of my aches and pains. My friend just let me talk. She listened to me talk my frustrations and worries out. She gave me the gift of listening.

God, she helped me realize that I have so many blessings to be thankful for. I can talk to you, and then

I turn over everything to your care. Lord, you make me feel whole as your presence washes over me. Thank you for giving me my family, friends, and most of all your compassion.

➣ Whom do you turn to when you have a problem?

_____

_____

_____

➣ Do you trust God? Why or why not?

_____

_____

_____

Tired

Hebrews 12:12–13 "So take a new grip with your tired hands and stand firm on your shaky legs. Mark out a straight path for your feet. Then those who follow you, though they are weak and lame, will not stumble and fall but will become strong."

I haven't felt well for at least a couple of months. I am so tired all of the time. I ache all over. I had better make an appointment with my doctor for a check up. I probably have a virus. I wake up tired and go to bed tired. It's getting hard just to keep up.

Jesus, in Scripture the sick came to you to be healed. You healed them all. Jesus, give me the wisdom to find out what is wrong with me. Give me the strength I need to take care of my family. Jesus, I trust you to help me.

➢ Have you ever been sick with out knowing why?

_____

_____

_____

➢ How did you cope with the not knowing?

_____

_____

_____

Exile

Ezekiel 20:41–42 "When I bring you home from exile, you will be as pleasing to me as an offering of perfumed incense. And I will display my holiness in you as all the nations watch."

I feel so alone in this world of choices. Every choice I seem to make is a wrong one, only because of my low self-confidence. I am afraid of making a mistake, yet I do so anyway.

God, I have the desire to turn my choice-making over to you, but I don't know how. Please lead me out of this exile of having low self-esteem brought on by this illness. I want to go back to the land of well-being and peace. Only with you will I make the right choices. I must stop talking in order to listen to you in the silence of my heart.

➣ Do you rely on the Lord when you have a choice to make? Why or why not?

_____

_____

_____

➣ Have you experienced an exile? What caused it?

_____

_____

_____

Worry

1 Peter 5:6–7 " … humble yourselves under the mighty power of God, and in his good time he will honor

you. Give all your worries and cares to God, for he cares about what happens to you."

I am worried about all the things I need to do, but I don't have the energy to get anything done. This concerns me because I don't seem to be getting any better. I have an appointment next week with Dr. Wilson for a check-up.

I am also concerned about my temper. I've flown off the handle at some of my family, and now they are not talking to me. I need to apologize to them because I lost control of my temper. I have been doing a lot of this lately

Oh, God, give me the strength I need to deal with everything. I am glad you are our constant companion and you care about us.

≽ Are you able to give all your worries over to God? Why or why not?

_____

_____

_____

≽ Do you feel that God cares about you? Why does he? Why doesn't he?

_____

_____

_____

Lazy

1 Thessalonians 1: 14 "Brothers and sisters, we urge you to warn those who are lazy. Encourage those who are timid. Take tender care of those who are weak. Be patient with everyone."

I am so disappointed in the way my aunt has treated me. I easily absorb the moods of others. I felt dumped on by Aunt Gertrude. She said she thought I was lazy and not paying attention to my family. She doesn't think I am ill at all.

Jesus, please comfort Aunt Gertrude. Bless her with a good mood. I know she is under stress, so please bring calmness to her heart. I need to learn to hand over to you the emotions of others. I only want to absorb your wonderful love into the quiet of my heart.

➤ Do you absorb people's moods?

_____

_____

_____

➤ Why? How can you avoid it?

_____

_____

_____

Tense

Hebrews 6:18–20 "Therefore, we who have fled to him for refuge can take new courage, for we can hold on to his promise with confidence. This confidence is like a strong and trustworthy anchor for our souls. It leads us through the curtain of heaven into God's inner sanctuary."

I am clinging tightly to my faith while I wait for the results of the physical tests I took. I am so confused, and I feel afraid. I thought that if I led a good life and loved you, I would be protected from harm. Now I don't feel well. It seems like I have a serious illness. I have no idea how to cope.

God, I will be quiet and listen for your inspiration. Yes, I know, you will help me by giving me the grace of a good attitude, a peaceful heart, and I will have a deeper faith. I will hold on to you as a boat is held with an anchor. I put my trust in you. You didn't say nothing bad would happen; you said, "I will never abandon you."

➤ Have you ever felt abandoned?

_____

_____

_____

_____

_____

_____

Stumble

Proverbs 3:21–26 "My child, don't lose sight of good planning and insight. Hang on to them, for they fill you with life and bring you honor and respect. They keep you safe on your way and keep your feet from stumbling. You can lie down without fear and enjoy pleasant dreams. You need not be afraid of disaster or the destruction that comes upon the wicked, for the Lord is your security. He will keep your foot from being caught in a trap."

I stumble all the time. I am clumsy and drop things on the floor and trip. The type of stumbling the verse means is my being prone to give into temptations. I put things off and wait to get it done tomorrow, and that is not good. Good planning and good insight do help me to keep from stumbling because I give myself goals that help me to know myself better.

I turn to you, God, to hear my prayer. I know that you are my security. I know that you will keep me from *stumbling in the dark. I open my eyes and ears, and I will follow the path you choose.*

> Have you ever stumbled?

_____

_____

_____

> How did God save you?

_____

_____

_____

Blessed

Luke 6:22 "God blesses you who are hated and excluded and mocked and cursed because you are identified with me, the Son of Man."

The problem is that people can only do so much. They are struggling themselves. As I go from day to day living with not feeling well, I feel empty and dry. It is hard to pray because I don't know what to pray for. The best thing to do is to be quiet, relax, and listen to God.

I long for you, God. I want you to reach out to me and comfort me. I am living in this gray landscape, and

I ask you to clear the grayness away. Put a rainbow over my cloudy landscape. Give me a feeling of peace.

➣ Do you trust others more than God?

_____

_____

_____

➣ What are some things God has done for you?

_____

_____

_____

STAGE 2: DIAGNOSIS

Anxious

Psalm 91:4 "He will shield you with his wings. He will shelter you with his feathers. His faithful promises are your armor and protection."

I need God's armor for protection. I feel threatened by the unknown. Things are very stressful at work. I was at the top of the list to be promoted, and another co-worker was promoted instead. The environment around me is so negative. I am also concerned about being sick and how much longer I will be able to keep my job.

God, I need your armor around me for a positive attitude. Life is so tiring. I am finding it hard to cope with disappointment and worry. God, please give me the grace of hope.

➣ When have you ever had to put on the armor of God?

_____

_____

_____

➣ Are you strong with God's power?

_____

_____

_____

Discouraged

Psalm 42:5–6 "Why am I discouraged? Why so sad? I will put my hope in God! I will praise him again—my Savior and my God!"

I am relying on my faith right now. Each new experience I go through brings me closer to God. I am so scared of the unknown. I have never had to deal with an illness before. I will have to learn all about the illness I can. I must give the unknown over to his care.

God, if I am scared, my family must be scared also. I must sit down with the family to talk about how this illness has and will affect each of us. We should keep everything out in the open for discussion. God, give us the grace to be calm and please give us your peace.

➤ Have you ever been faced with something that is not in your control?

_____

_____

_____

➤ Did you hand the problem over to God's wisdom?

_____

_____

_____

Reliance

Mark 4:40 "And he asked them, 'Why are you so afraid? Do you still not have faith in me?'"

I no longer know what my faith is. I am very perplexed. Is God really with me? I feel very empty. I fear that my once positive attitude has been replaced by a spirit of grayness. I can't concentrate. I can't read. I can't comprehend anything. I realize that the news that I received from the doctor about my condition has been hard on all of us. I have an illness that will get progressively worse. There is no cure.

God, please clear out the fog in my heart. Give me the faith to know that you are with us. Bind up my ill-

ness with your love. Breathe your Holy Spirit back into my heart.

➤ Are you ever afraid?

_____

_____

_____

➤ Do you hand over your fear to God? If not, why?

_____

_____

_____

Confidence

Psalm 13:5–6 "I trust in your unfailing love. I will rejoice because you have rescued me.

I will sing to the Lord because he has been so good to me."

God has been good to me. I do feel free from the power of sin except for one thing: I have a lack of trust that everything will be okay. I haven't been feeling well lately. At first my doctor discounted my symptoms saying I was fine. I felt so vulnerable. I feared that I was going to be left alone in pain. Well, I did get worse, and my doctor told me that I do have a chronic illness. That I was just going to have to live with it. With God's guidance, we will be fine.

God, I was relieved to finally find out what is wrong. I can accept my fate, because you give me the strength I need. I know you are with me. I love you, God. Please bring peace to my family.

➤ Have you ever been left waiting for news?

_____

_____

_____

➤ Did you pray for patience?

_____

_____

_____

Drained

Psalm 77:3 "All night long I pray, with hands lifted toward heaven, pleading. There can be no joy for me until he acts. I think of God, and I moan, overwhelmed with longing for his help."

I am longing to feel God's presence once again in my life. God seems so far away. The tests have showed my illness is indeed chronic, and it is hard to adjust to the results. I find that I deny that I am sick until the symptoms hit once again. I will just have to face it and learn to live it. My life is drained of all peace. My heart is aching. All I am doing is crying. I can't eat or sleep.

God, please hear my cry. Place into my heart new life and new dreams. I can't do this by myself. I need to be strong, not only for myself but for my loved ones. I need your grace. Already I feel your peace washing over me.

➣ Have you ever longed for God's presence?

_____

_____

_____

➣ What happened?

_____

_____

_____

Grace

Romans 1:7 "May grace and peace be yours from God our Father and the Lord Jesus Christ."

I know the answer to my feeling sick, and I don't like it. It took a long while of waiting for the doctor to come up with the answer, which is hard on all of us. Now that we know, I ask Jesus to give me the grace to endure what is ahead. I am in shock that my body is letting me down. I will never be healthy again. My poor family will have to deal with me.

Jesus, the answer is in you. We need your grace to encourage us to overcome our natural tendencies for negative thinking. Give us positive thoughts as we cope with this illness that will affect us all.

➢ Is your natural tendency to be negative?

_____

_____

_____

➢ Does it help you?

_____

_____

_____

Stage 3: Anger

Questioning

Acts 15:10–11 "Why are you now questioning God's way by burdening the Gentile believers with a yoke that neither we nor our ancestors were able to bear? We believe that we are all saved the same way, by the special favor of the Lord Jesus."

Jesus gave his life so that we could be saved from the evil that is in the world. All we have to do is follow him. It sounds so simple, but following him is a hard thing for us to do because there are so many distractions. My low self-esteem puts up a wall of distortion that keeps me from following him. Instead I wallow in my illness and I wonder what I did to deserve being ill. I answer myself back, "Why not?"

Jesus, I must say, though, that because of my strong foundation of faith, you do break through my low self-esteem. You bring hope out of my sadness. Deep down in my heart there is a longing to be in relationship with you.

➢ Have you ever felt like a sheep?

_____

_____

_____

➢ Has someone ever condemned you?

_____

_____

_____

Demands

1 Thessalonians 2:6–8 "As apostles of Christ we certainly had a right to make some demands of you, but we were as gentle among you as a mother feeding and caring for her own children. We loved you so much that we gave you not only God's Good News but our own lives, too."

I am in the core of a whirlwind of demands by everyone around me. I want to please people and I want to be a good Christian by putting others before myself. As time goes on I am becoming filled with resentment. I am tired of their demands. I want to strike out at everyone. On top of everything, I don't feel well and I am tired.

Jesus, I am trying to follow your teachings but perhaps I don't really understand them. I am trying to live up to the expectations of others instead of truly loving them. I need to be quiet so I can listen to your wisdom. I need you to guide me along the true path of Christian love. Thank you, Jesus.

➤ Have you ever felt resentment toward others?

_____

_____

_____

➤ Did you go to God for guidance?

_____

_____

_____

Storm

Psalm 5:11 "But let all who take refuge in you rejoice; let them sing joyful praises forever. Protect them, so all who love your name may be filled with joy."

God is my refuge in a storm; life is banging at

the door of my heart. I am in the midst off a storm. I feel okay one minute, yet I feel a deep fear the next. All of my defenses to cope with my illness are being battered away, leaving my emotion raw. It is hard to get the energy to do what used to be so easy for me. I am so stiff, and I ache. The medication helps, but I have good days and bad days when I don't feel like moving.

God, consol and protect me. Give me courage as I walk through this storm of having a chronic illness. Bless my loved ones and reassure them that I do appreciate all they are doing for me.

➣ Have you ever had to depend on others to do things for you?

_____

_____

_____

➣ How did being dependent make you feel?

_____

_____

_____

Hurt

Luke 6:28–29 "Pray for the happiness of those who curse you. Pray for those who hurt you."

I contemplate that pain and suffering have a way of getting our attention. Sometimes it brings us to our knees. If we feel remorse about something we have done, we will want to change our ways. We are hurt and we don't want to hurt anymore. We ask Jesus to save us from ourselves.

Jesus, lift me up to your healing. Free me from my pain of guilt. I have been so impatient with this illness. I get tired of having to ask for help around the house. I am mad that I have to stay at home or at the office. I am too tired to go anywhere else. I am being selfish. You heal and give me the strength to endure. I ask for your peace.

➢ Have you experienced pain?

_____

_____

_____

➢ What did you do about it?

_____

_____

_____

Encouragement

1 Thessalonians 5:14 "Encourage those who are timid. Take tender care of those who are weak. Be patient with everyone."

I have been extremely irritable because I have been worried about my health. I am tired because I'm not sleeping well at night. When I feel like this, I tend to dump on others. I don't have any patience. I hate waiting in line; I experience driver's rage; I feel like yelling and screaming.

Jesus, please send your Spirit to soothe my soul. I need your help to love others with brotherly love. Help me be a source of encouragement for others. Most of all, help me to be patient.

➣ Do you give encouragement to others?

_____

_____

_____

➣ Are you a patient person?

_____

_____

_____

Forgive

Psalm 86:5–7 "O Lord, you are so good, so ready to forgive, so full of unfailing love for all who ask your aid. Listen closely to my prayer, O Lord; hear my urgent cry. I will call to you whenever trouble strikes, and you will answer me."

Jesus brings forgiveness. I need his help in forgiving myself for not behaving very well. Because I wasn't feeling in good health, I lost my temper. I was completely out of control. I said a number of things to the people in my Scripture Study Group that I shouldn't have said. I have apologized and asked them to forgive me, but I know I betrayed a special bond of trust that I had with them. The damage is done.

Jesus, please help me accept the harm I have done, learn from it, and then move on. Because I don't feel good and that makes me irritable is no excuse for losing control. Help me be thoughtful, patient, and calm.

➣ Have you ever lost a friend because you lost your temper?

_____

_____

_____

➤ What drives you to anger in those instances?

_____

_____

_____

Bitterness

Ephesians 5:31–32 "Get rid of all bitterness, rage, anger, harsh words, and slander, as well as all types of malicious behavior. Instead, be kind to each other, tenderhearted, forgiving one another, just as God through Christ has forgiven you."

At times during my illness, I have been bitter, angry, and have said some very hurtful things. I felt like striking out at everyone. Then it dawned on me that I needed to talk to God about my bitterness. Why was I feeling bitter when I had much to be thankful for? Who wants to be around someone who is always in a bad mood? I certainly don't want to be around someone who is grouchy.

God, help me to be kind to those around me. When I am hurt by something they say or do, help me forgive them as well as myself. Only through your grace can I find peace.

➤ Have you ever been bitter about something?

_____

_____

_____

➤ Did bitterness take away your anger?

_____

_____

_____

Stage 4: Depression

Pain

1 Peter 4:1 "So then, since Christ suffered physical pain, you must arm yourselves with the same attitude he had, and be ready to suffer, too. For if you are willing to suffer for Christ, you have decided to stop sinning."

Jesus suffered while he was here on earth. Just like I do, he prayed and he pleaded and cried to God who could have saved him from his suffering and his impending death. Even though Jesus was the son of God, he learned about obedience from the things he suffered. This is the way God was able to qualify Jesus as a perfect high priest. Jesus is the source of salvation for eternity for all who obey him.

Dear God, you sometimes ask us to do the impossible. You always have a reason, although we don't always understand it. You asked Jesus to do a very hard thing. Jesus obeyed God. He became a bridge from us to you through his death and resurrection.

⮞ Do you feel that Jesus understands our suffering?

_____

_____

_____

⮞ How did God qualify Jesus as a high priest?

_____

_____

_____

Love

Psalm 66:20 "Praise God, who did not ignore my prayer and did not withdraw his unfailing love from me."

God listens to my prayer. Often I run into people who turn away from me when I am talking. It makes me feel discounted. When I am ignored in this way, I know that my voice is soft and I don't speak plainly. I begin doubting myself. I feel very self-conscious.

God, how can I make people listen to me like you listen to my prayers? I need to listen to your wisdom. I need to talk a little louder and make people hear me.

➢ How do you attract people's attention?

_____

_____

_____

➢ Have you ever felt ignored?

_____

_____

_____

Desert

Psalm 44:18–19 "We have not strayed from your path. Yet you have crushed us in the desert. You have covered us with darkness and death."

I really need to depend on God. I need his help in understanding the situation I am in. I don't think I can bear the burden that I am carrying now. I feel drained and all my joy seems to be gone. My body feels like a dried carcass blowing in the wind. A carcass that is forgotten, alone. Ever since I have been sick, I have only the memory of what once was.

Father, please protect me from this arid desert I am

in. Bring the fresh rain of your grace to my heart. Lift my spirit so that I may soar with the freedom your love brings to me.

➤ Have you ever been in a desert?

_____

_____

_____

➤ What did it feel like?

_____

_____

_____

Pride

Proverbs 11:2 "Pride leads to disgrace, but with humility comes wisdom."

There was a time not so long ago when I was very smug about my life. I had everything I wanted. I knew it all. People would tell me to stop being so smug. Life caught up with me and the rug was pulled out from under me. Instead of the pride I once had, I felt reticent. My life was forever changed by this illness that would go on and on.

Lord, I beg you to help me find something I can do. I want to be productive again. Help me to be patient and kind. Take away this sadness from my heart. I know you are with me.

➤ Have you ever had too much pride?

_____

_____

_____

➤ Have you ever been reticent?

_____

_____

_____

Quiet

1 Corinthians 4:21 "Which do you choose? Should I come with punishment and scolding, or should I come with quiet love and gentleness?"

I want to pray for my boss. I dread going to work because he is always ranting and raving about some thing or other. Just being in his loud presence sends my stomach churning and my anxiety level up. When I get home I can't calm down.

Father, I need quiet. I turn to you for peace. I am so exhausted. This isn't good for my health. Please bless my boss. By asking for your blessing of my boss, I will feel free from resentment, and I will be able to forgive him.

> ➣ How do protect yourself from loud and crude people?

_____

_____

_____

> ➣ Do you need quiet time?

_____

_____

_____

Unique

James 3:17 "But the wisdom that comes from heaven is first of all pure. It is also peace loving, gentle at all times and willing to yield to others. It is full of mercy and good deeds."

My main fault in life is that I am not willing to yield to others' points of view. If my point of view is rejected, I feel rejected. Now that I am sick, I become sad when others disagree with me. I don't cope very well.

Father, give me your wisdom. Help me to be a loving,

courteous person. You made each of us to be unique. We serve you in our own individual way, in a community of believers coming together for the common cause to love you.

➣ In what ways are you unique?

_____

_____

_____

➣ Do you appreciate the uniqueness of others?

_____

_____

_____

Patience

James 5:10–11 "For examples of patience in suffering, dear brothers and sisters, look at the prophets who spoke in the name of the Lord. We give great honor to those who endure under suffering. Job is an example of a man who endured patiently. From his experience we see how the Lord's plan finally ended in good, for he is full of tenderness and mercy."

I am in need of patience right now. God promises peace and joy in the midst of suffering. I need to listen to God in my heart, but that is easier said than done. My life seems to be falling apart, and my dreams have broken down. I have this illness that my family and I have to live with. Things have changed so much and there are no answers.

Lord, I ask you to shine your light of wisdom on us. Please give me the grace to change my negative attitude to a positive one. God, I am grateful to you no matter what is going on in my life.

➢ Are you grateful to God for his blessings?

_____

_____

_____

➢ Do you have the patience to endure life's trials?

_____

_____

_____

Fear

Psalm 46:2–3 "So we will not fear, even if earthquakes come and the mountains crumble into the sea. Let the oceans roar and foam. Let the mountains tremble as the waters surge!"

I ask for freedom from all of my fears. I spend

my days worrying about all kinds of things. If I do have a moment when there is nothing to worry about, I—without thinking—look for something I can worry about. It seems like I am not comfortable unless I worry about something. Of course my illness does give me continual fear and worry. Over a period of time this negative thinking will break me down.

God, help me break free from this negative thinking. This is damaging my peace of mind. Disconnect these tangled lines of fear and put one straight line to my heart with positive thinking. Thank you.

➤ What do you fear?

_____

_____

_____

➤ Have you prayed about it?

_____

_____

_____

Family

1 Timothy 3:4 "He must manage his own family well, with children who respect and obey him."

I realize that we must manage our own family well. As of late being sick and all I haven't wanted to be around anyone. That's not fair to them. I certainly haven't been managing them at all. I have been isolated because I don't have the energy to interact with anyone.

Father, I beg of you to help me listen to your wisdom. Open my mind to the sunlight of your love. Allow the light to filter to every pore of my body. Bring healing to my sad soul. Show me how to manage my family and help them to manage me.

➤ How is your family managed?

_____

_____

_____

➤ Do you listen to God's wisdom?

_____

_____

_____

Stage 5: Coping

Distress

Psalm 107:6–7 "'Lord, help!' they cried in their trouble, and he rescued them from their distress."

I need God's encouragement. The work I try to do at work is always wrong. Yesterday at the office I put together a report on what I had read, and the office shared the reading of reports with each other before printing them. My boss told me that I didn't follow directions … besides that, I had missed the point. He said he had trusted me to use the correct information, but it appeared he would not be able to trust me again.

God, I am so hurt. Help me to be focused and not distracted by not feeling well. But I need your aid. Help me to trust myself again. Bless my boss. I do want to forgive him.

> ⮞ What was your most embarrassing moment?

_____

_____

_____

> ⮞ How did you react?

_____

_____

_____

Gloomy

Job 30:3 "They are gaunt with hunger and flee to the deserts and the wastelands, desolate and gloomy."

My attitude is so very gloomy without a ray of light to boost it. Each day seems to bring new problems added to old problems. I am weighed down by all of these burdens. I am so tired; I am restless and can't relax. I am worried about how under-the-weather I feel. My coping skills are depleted.

God, I need to focus on what is going well. My family and friends are real blessings to me. All will be well.

Thank you for turning me from a gloomy attitude to an encouraging one.

➤ Have you ever been pessimistic?

_____

_____

_____

➤ Did praying bring you encouragement?

_____

_____

_____

Afraid

Acts 18:9 "Don't be afraid! Speak out! Don't be silent! For I am with you, and no one will harm you because many people here in this city belong to me."

I must be pretty hard to deal with right now. I am very fearful that nothing will get any better. I don't see anything in a positive light. I try to be strong and handle everything by myself. I have not often asked for anything God didn't know already. I figured he knew I was discouraged, so I wouldn't be telling him anything new.

God, I can see the folly of not turning to you early on. I didn't realize the importance of verbalizing my feelings to you. It is important to verbalize so I can listen to

*myself. I turn to you for help that is already being given
to me by you.*

➣ Are you able to verbalize your feelings to
God?

_____

_____

_____

➣ Does God already know how hurt you are
feeling?

_____

_____

_____

Agreement

Proverbs 6:2–3 "... if you have trapped yourself by
your agreement and are caught by what you said—
quick, get out of it if you possibly can! You have
placed yourself at your friend's mercy."

I would give just about everything to be well
again. I would promise God I would do all the reli-
gious practices in the world. I would promise him
that I would be a better person. No matter if I am

sick or not, I should do all these things any way. I should not try to bargain with him.

God, I would like to be well again, but I realize that I can do many things for you through my illness. All I ask is that you help my family adjust to my illness. It is hard on them. Thank you.

➣ Have you ever bargained with the Lord?

_____
_____
_____

➣ What happened?

_____
_____
_____

Control

Psalm 5:3 "Listen to my voice in the morning, Lord. Each morning I bring my requests to you and wait expectantly."

I need to learn that I should listen to God. I am so busy telling him how to fix my illness that I don't take time to listen to him. My prayers are nothing other than giving God instructions as to how my life should be. When my life is hit by an obstacle, I become angry at him for not following my instructions.

God, please free me from this need to control. Help me trust your ways and not my ways. Help me have a listening heart. It is one thing to take responsibility for myself, but I need to also let go and trust you.

➤ Why do you tell God what to do?

_____

_____

_____

➤ How can you let go and let God?

_____

_____

_____

Hope

Psalm 31:24 "So be strong and take courage, all you who put your hope in the Lord!"

I long for the day when my heart-filled emotion of emptiness will be filled with hope. I go from one thing to another. I go around in circles getting nothing done. I yearn for your peace, yet all I feel is the nagging feeling of restlessness. I must learn to cope with my illness and learn new ways of getting things done.

God, help me surrender my life to your ways. Help me live in the present moment.

Strip everything away out of my mind that tears me away from your wisdom. Turn my grief into a source of joy and hope.

➣ Do you live in the present moment?

_____

_____

_____

➣ Are you able to surrender your hopes and dreams to God's control?

_____

_____

_____

Helpless

Psalm 71:17–18 "O God, you have taught me from my earliest childhood, and I have constantly told others about the wonderful things you do. Now that I am old and gray, do not abandon me, O God."

God has been with me all of my life. I beg him to give me the courage I need as my body breaks down.

Being sick is being vulnerable in a society that thinks we are in complete control of own destiny. When something goes wrong, we find someone or something to blame it on. Yet when we get a sickness that is chronic, we learn that we humans are not in control of anything at all.

God, when I was a vulnerable child, you did give me strength as I sat in prayer in your house of worship. I felt safe as you replaced my fears with hope and courage. I now sit before you, once again vulnerable, and I ask that you replace my fears with hope and courage.

➤ Have you ever felt vulnerable?

_____

_____

_____

➤ Did you pray for hope and courage?

_____

_____

_____

Path
Psalm 25:4–5 "Show me the path where I should walk, O Lord; point out the right road for me to follow.

Lead me by your truth and teach me, for you are the God who saves me. All day long I put my hope in you."

I have come to a fork in the road of my spiritual journey. Making the decision of which way I should go is confusing. I am a creature of habit, so when life changes come about I either face them with courage or else fear. I am sick. I have to learn to adjust to it.

God, I turn to you asking for the courage to face life with my illness. When I feel fearful, guide me to a feeling that all will be well. I know that you are with me, and I thank you.

➢ What makes you feel fearful?

_____

_____

_____

➢ Do you ask for God's wisdom?

_____

_____

_____

STAGE 6:
ACCEPTANCE AND HOPE

Help

1 Peter 4:11 "Are you called to help others? Do it with all the strength and energy that God supplies. Then God will be given glory in everything through Jesus Christ. All glory and power belong to him forever and ever. Amen."

I am turning to Christ more and more everyday because I receive strength and comfort from him. Perhaps my health doesn't change, but my attitude changes. I certainly do grow. No one wants suffering to come into their lives, but sure enough it does in one form or another. Why is it for our benefit and salvation? We learn from suffering that we don't have

control. Only God controls and gives us encouragement to endure.

*God, I've gotten to the point of realizing that I need
to hand all my problems over to your care. I can hand my
burdens over to you with relief. To find peace I need to
trust in you. Thank you, God, for your comfort.*

➢ How are you able to give encouragement to
others?

_____

_____

_____

➢ How are you able to cope with problems?

_____

_____

_____

Love

1 Corinthians 13:13 "There are three things that will
endure—faith, hope, and love—and the greatest of
these is love."

I lean on God's grace to help me to feel hopeful.
Things have been down for me lately. I have been in
a negative state of mind. I have been worried about

my health. The worry almost overcomes me and it is hard to function.

God, please give me the wisdom to know how to cope with my illness. I know it is a chronic and not a life-threatening illness. I will have good days and bad days when I will need help. Faith and hope are important, but love is the most important and is the greatest. I do love my family and friends, and I love you. All will be well.

➢ Do you have hope?

_____

_____

_____

➢ Do you feel that you endure so long as you have God's love?

_____

_____

_____

Mercy

Luke 10:37 "The man replied, 'The one who showed him mercy.' Then Jesus said, 'Yes, now go and do the same.'"

These past months have been very hard to bear.

My emotions have been raw. The only relief from worry has been sleeping. Then I wake up and realize once again that I am ill. I have to learn to adjust to the fact that it is chronic and I am going to have to live with it.

Father, I have been pouring my heart out to you. A feeling of steadiness is beginning to grow in my soul. I hear a whispering of your reassurance and love coming deep within. I am beginning to have hope. I know that you do listen to me and you are showering your mercy on me. Thank you, God.

➤ When has God shown his mercy to you?

_____

_____

_____

➤ Do you feel that God listens to you?

_____

_____

_____

Good

Ephesians 4:29 "Let everything you say be good and helpful, so that your words will be an encouragement to those who hear them."

I need to give encouragement to others. I am a perfectionist. I want everything to be in perfect order. My perfectionism causes me to be highly critical of how people do things, and I let them know it. Of course they back away. Can't say I blame them.

God, please heal me of this critical perfectionism I have. Lately because of my chronic illness I have been anxious to the point of not wanting to do anything. I don't even want to be around anyone. I place this anxiety and perfectionism into your hands. I pray that with your help, I will live each day with the sense that all is well no matter what is happening.

➤ Do you live each day with sense that all is well?

_____
_____
_____

➤ Are you a perfectionist?

_____
_____
_____

Unconditional
Luke 10:16 "Then he said to the disciples, 'Anyone

who accepts your message is also accepting me. And anyone who rejects you is rejecting me. And anyone who rejects me is rejecting God who sent me.'"

I look for kindness and truth in the world. Sometimes I find it, but most of the time I don't. The world's love is conditional, but God's love is unconditional. I only receive this type love from him.

God, help me to feel deep within my heart that I am constantly receiving the blessings of your love and truth. Help me give to others the unconditional love I want that they can't readily give. Through my illness give me a big heart that is filled with understanding and compassion.

➣ Do you have compassion for others who are in need?

_____

_____

_____

➣ Name the people who have been kind to you.

_____

_____

_____

Accept

Mark 4:18–19 "The thorny ground represents those who hear and accept the Good News, but all too quickly the message is crowded out by the cares of this life, the lure of wealth, and the desire for nice things."

I was on the path of loving the lures of the world. I wanted to have nice things. I wanted my children to be smart, so I pushed them to the point that they didn't want to go to school. Now that I am sick I don't even want to have the things the world offers. My children no longer have to be perfect. I want them to be good people instead.

God, I love you. By being blind-sided with this illness, I have the time to see where I was going wrong in my attitude. I have had to let go of my dreams, and I must dream new dreams. Yes, I think I'm accepting this life change by having a positive attitude. I ask you, God, to continue to give me life-giving positive attitudes.

➤ What would you never want to give up?

_____

_____

_____

➣ How do you go about adjusting to change?

_____

_____

_____

Hospitality

Luke 10:7 "Don't hesitate to accept hospitality, because those who work deserve their pay."

At the beginning of this illness, I just wanted to be alone. There seemed so much to think about. I became isolated. I refused all invitations except going to work, and even there I kept to myself. That was bad for me and bad for my family too.

God, I have now become more outgoing. The house is a happy place since we laugh again. Yes, indeed, when I saw the funny side of life again, I knew I was adjusting to the fact that I have a chronic illness. I am ready to dream new dreams. God is at my side.

➣ What are your dreams?

_____

_____

_____

➤ Is God at your side?

_____

_____

_____

Mystery

Matthew 9:35–38 "Jesus traveled through all the cities and villages of that area, teaching in the synagogues and announcing the Good News about the Kingdom. And wherever he went, he healed people of every sort of disease and illness. He felt great pity for the crowds that came, because their problems were so great and they didn't know where to go for help. They were like sheep without a shepherd."

It is a mystery why Jesus heals people in different ways. Some are healed physically, some emotionally, others spiritually. Some are given the grace of strength and courage to cope. Others are used by God to reach out with empathy. It doesn't appear that I will be physically healed, so I want to be spiritually healed; therefore, I will spend time reading the Scriptures and join the crowds that are following Jesus.

God, give me courage to face my illness head-on. You have given me so many blessings, the best being the faith *my family and I have. May we always have positive attitudes.*

➣ What blessings has God given you?

_____

_____

_____

➣ What positive thing can you do with these blessings?

_____

_____

_____

Food For Thought

Life

Relax your body—Slow your breathing—
Relax in God's presence.
God made my lungs—I breathe in his
love—In thanks and love I am alive.

Isaiah 40:6–8 "A voice said, 'Shout!' I asked, 'What should I shout?' 'Shout that people are like the grass that dies away. Their beauty fades as quickly as the beauty of flowers in a field. The grass withers, and the flowers fade beneath the breath of the Lord. And so it is with people. The grass withers, and the flowers fade, but the word of our God stands forever.'"

Think about the fact that we are in this world for a short time. How does this thought make you feel?

What do you believe God wants you to accomplish during this short time on earth? What has God given you to face life with strength and courage? In what ways has God given you his love and comfort?

_____

_____

_____

_____

_____

_____

Father, I pray that I will live my life in your light. In order do so, I ask you to give me blessings of your courage and strength. I am so fragile, but with your help, I can become whole, reflecting your love and your word. Amen

Enemies

Become comfortable—Calm your inner
spirit—Rest quietly in presence of God

Psalm 31:1–2 "O Lord, I have come to you for protection; don't let me be put to shame. Rescue me, for you always do what is right. Bend down and listen to me; rescue me quickly. Be for me a great rock of safety, a fortress where my enemies cannot reach me."

What kind of enemies could defeat me? I don't have any enemies, do I? Does this apply to something deep inside of me? I really am my own worse enemy when I am hard on myself and when I drive myself for a perfection that just isn't there. Am I my own worse enemy when I insist living my life on my own without asking God for help and guidance? When I ignore trying to have a relationship with the Lord and when I fail to accept his unconditional love, I am my own worse enemy.

_____

_____

_____

_____

_____

_____

Lord, you give me your unconditional love to accept through your healing grace. Help me remember to turn my burdens over to your care as you walk by my side on this my journey. Amen

Rejection

Get comfortable—Relax any tension you
may be feeling—Slow your breathing
Relax your body—Relax your mind—
God is present in your heart
Isaiah 53:7 "He was oppressed and treated harshly, yet

he never said a word. He was led as a lamb to the slaughter. And as a sheep is silent before the shearers, he did not open his mouth."

Think about Jesus, the Son of God, not being accepted in the world. How do I feel when people don't accept me? What is my reaction? Do I turn to the Lord? Or do I strike out in anger? Do I believe that Jesus truly understands how I feel during these times of feeling rejected by others? Do I believe that God will give me the strength and courage to overcome this feeling of rejection? Does rejection bring spiritual growth?

_____

_____

_____

_____

_____

_____

Jesus, with your loving help, I know that my self worth comes from your unconditional love for me. I give you all my feelings of rejection. I seek to live in peaceful joy. Amen

Compassion
Make yourself comfortable—
Breathe deeply—Inhale the presence of God
I live in you—You are deep within my heart—
I love you, God

John 15:12 "I command you to love each other in the same way that I love you."

How much does God love me? Do I believe that God is compassionate toward me? What does the word *compassionate* mean? Does it mean to suffer with? Does God suffer with me in my everyday problems, hurts, confusion, questions, and struggles? I pray that I am a compassionate person. I want to be there for people whenever I can. Am I able to love others as much as God loves me?

_____

_____

_____

_____

_____

_____

Lord of my heart, help me to have a compassionate heart. Give me the grace to love others as much as you love me. Amen

Competition

Breathe in—Breathe out—Breathe slowly

God, I am your creation—You chose me to live for you

Peter 1:2–3 "May God bless you with his special favor and wonderful peace as you come to know Jesus, our God and Lord, better and better. As we know Jesus better, his divine power gives us everything we need for living a godly life."

What hinders me from feeling God's kindness and peace? Do I ever find myself trying to live up to the world's view of living life to the fullest? Do I compare myself with others? Does this type of competition help me feel love toward others? Do I believe that God loves me unconditionally? Do I want more and more of God's kindness and peace?

_____

_____

_____

_____

_____

_____

Lord, I need your guidance for living a peaceful life in the midst of the competition of the world. Free me from everything that hinders me from receiving your kindness and peace. Amen.

Lost

Breathe in the air around you—Breathe
out tension—Relax your shoulders

Relax your arms—*I love you, Lord, with all my heart*
Ezekiel 34:3–31 "In this way, they will know that I, the Lord, their God, am with them. And they will know that they, the people of Israel, are my people, says the Sovereign Lord. You are my flock, the sheep of my pasture. You are my people, and I am your God, says the Sovereign Lord."

Think of a pasture filled with a flock of sheep. Jesus the Good Shepherd is taking care of these vulnerable sheep. One of the little lambs gets separated from the flock and becomes confused and lost. Have you ever felt lost and confused in the pasture of life? What does Jesus the Good Shepherd do? Does he lead you like the little lost lamb back to safety? Were you aware that you were being led to safety? Listen to Jesus the Good Shepherd speaking to you in the peaceful silence of your heart.

_____

_____

_____

_____

_____

_____

Jesus, protect me from being led astray in this pasture of life. I put my being into your loving care. Amen

Abandon

Matthew 5:45–46 "In that way, you will be acting as true children of your Father in heaven. For he gives his sunlight to both the evil and the good, and he sends rain on the just and on the unjust, too."

Living in this world is dangerous for our bodies as well as our souls. We face temptations and bad health as well happiness too. I would hate to face this world without having God's wisdom, guidance, and presence in my life. It's wonderful knowing that God has promised he would never abandon us.

_____

_____

_____

_____

_____

God, you didn't promise us a rose garden. You knew that life would have some rough spots along the way. You are with us to share the good as well as the bad times with us.

Thank you, God.

ENDNOTE

1. Encarta ® World English Dictionary © & (P) 1998–2005 Microsoft Corporation. All rights reserved.

Another book by Donna:

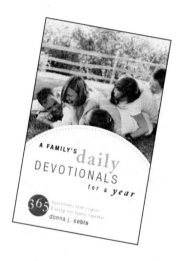

A Family's Daily Devotionals for a Year
a book for the entire family, and available at
www.tatepublishing.com.

Visit Donna at her web site, www.donnajcoble.
com.

listen|imagine|view|experience

AUDIO BOOK DOWNLOAD INCLUDED WITH THIS BOOK!

In your hands you hold a complete digital entertainment package. Besides purchasing the paper version of this book, this book includes a free download of the audio version of this book. Simply use the code listed below when visiting our website. Once downloaded to your computer, you can listen to the book through your computer's speakers, burn it to an audio CD or save the file to your portable music device (such as Apple's popular iPod) and listen on the go!

How to get your free audio book digital download:

1. Visit www.tatepublishing.com and click on the e|LIVE logo on the home page.
2. Enter the following coupon code:
   7ad4-4ebd-ed87-cb46-d94a-9ba9-bd76-24dc
   Download the audio book from your e|LIVE digital locker and begin enjoying your new digital entertainment package today!